OIT RULES!!

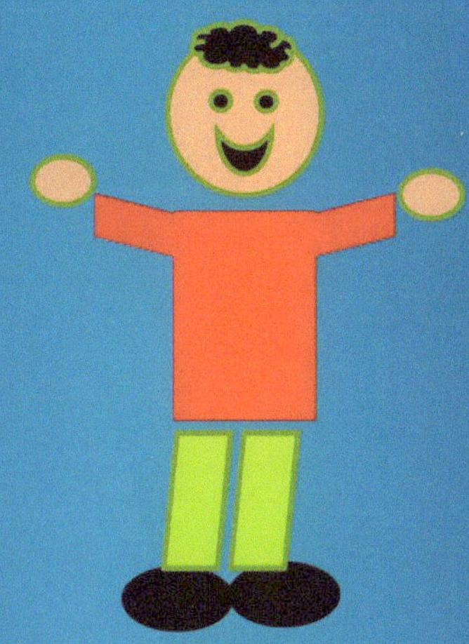

By Dr. Lilly-Rose Paraskevas

OIT Rules!

BY DR LILLY-ROSE PARASKEVAS

Note for the parents-

- This book was put together not to recommend oral immunotherapy or to suggest it is a cure for all food allergies but, once you have made the decision to pursue this treatment, to help your little ones understand the process of oral immunotherapy and all the new rules they must follow in order to go through the process

- Oral immunotherapy is always done under close supervision of an allergist who specializes in this procedure

- This book is for informational purposes only and is in no way a replacement for medical advice or a replacement for the instructions provided to you by your allergist with whom you are undergoing oral immunotherapy. By reading this book, you are not establishing a doctor-patient relationship with any physician.

- The content in the book is based on the current state of medical information as of the time the book was written, so check with your allergist for the most up-to-date advice

- If any content in this book contradicts or differs from advice provided by your allergist, you likely should follow the advice of your allergist, who has specific knowledge regarding your child's medical condition

- Do not ever delay seeking treatment because of something you read in this book

- I provided areas where you can personalize the book for the unique needs of your child; feel free to add in his or her own specific instructions so your child can use this book as a guide through the oral immunotherapy journey

- It was my goal to give our children a book that makes them feel represented and gives them a sense of control over their own treatment and health.

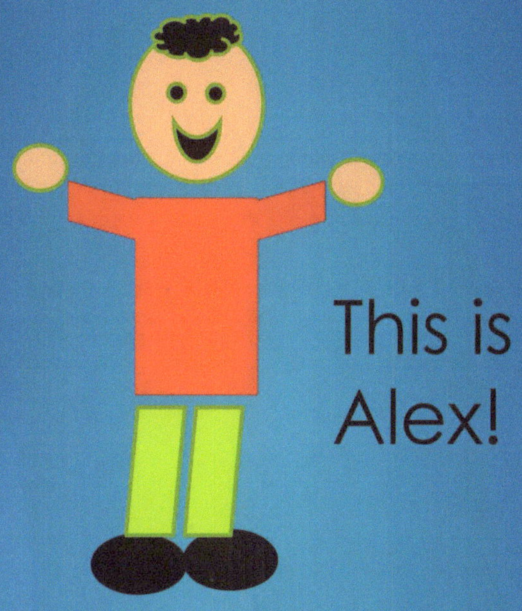

This is
Alex!

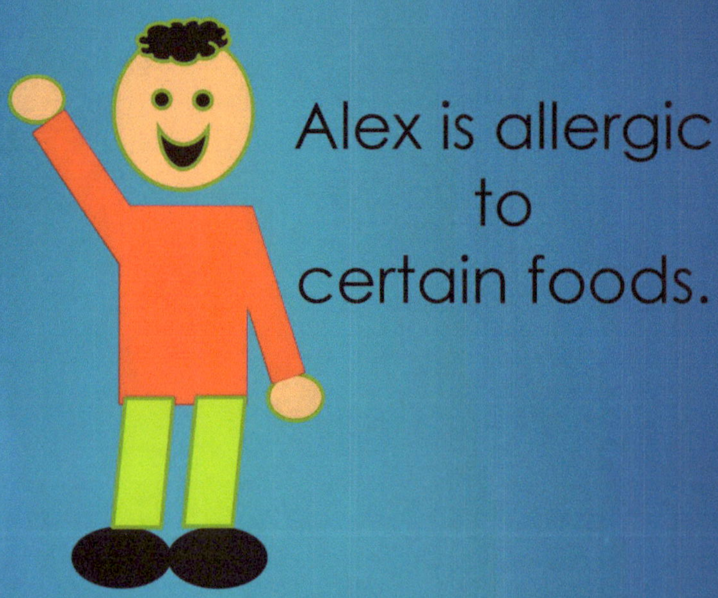

Alex is allergic
to
certain foods.

Alex is allergic to:
(circle all that apply)

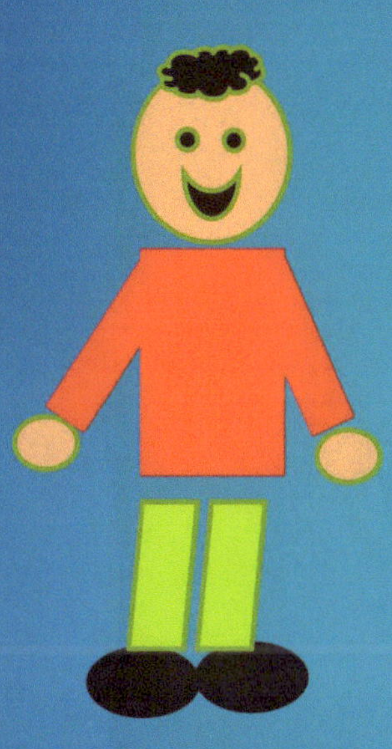

- **Cow's milk (dairy)**
- **Soy**
- **Eggs**
- **Nuts**
- **Wheat**
- **Peanuts**
- **Fish**
- **Shellfish**
- **Sesame**

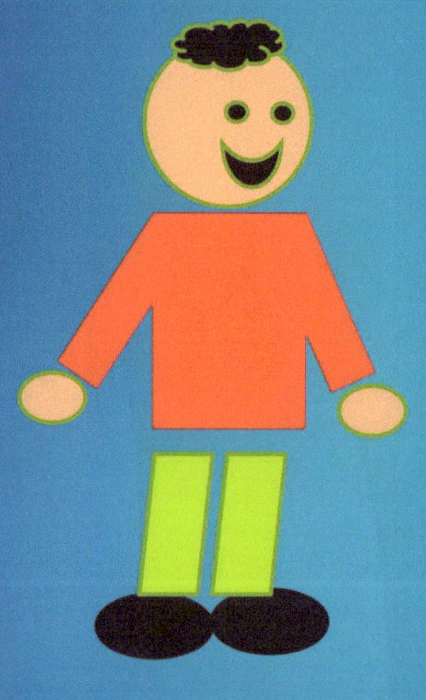

When a
person is
allergic to a
food,
it means that
his immune
system thinks
it's bad for
him.

Our immune system inside our bodies protects us from getting sick by fighting harmful germs.

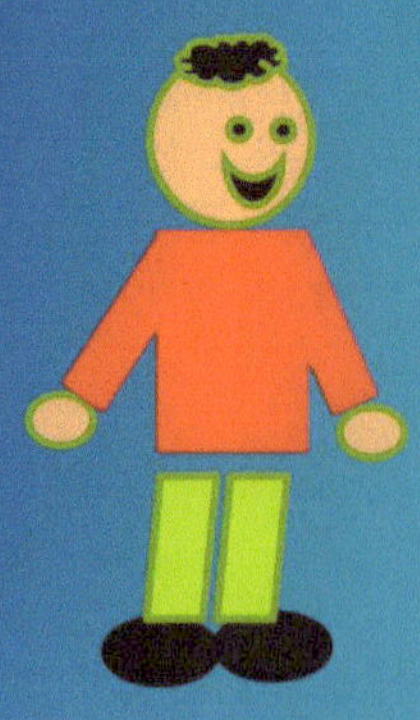

But in this case, Alex's immune system thinks the FOOD is bad for him. So whenever he eats it, or sometimes even TOUCHES it, he gets sick

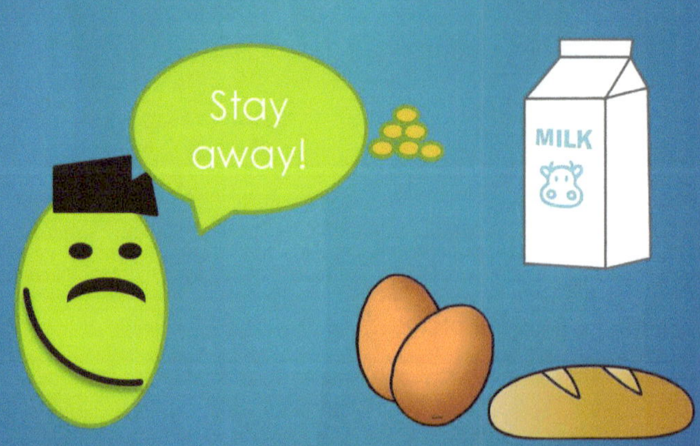

He has to be careful
that anything he eats
has not touched
anything that he is
allergic to.

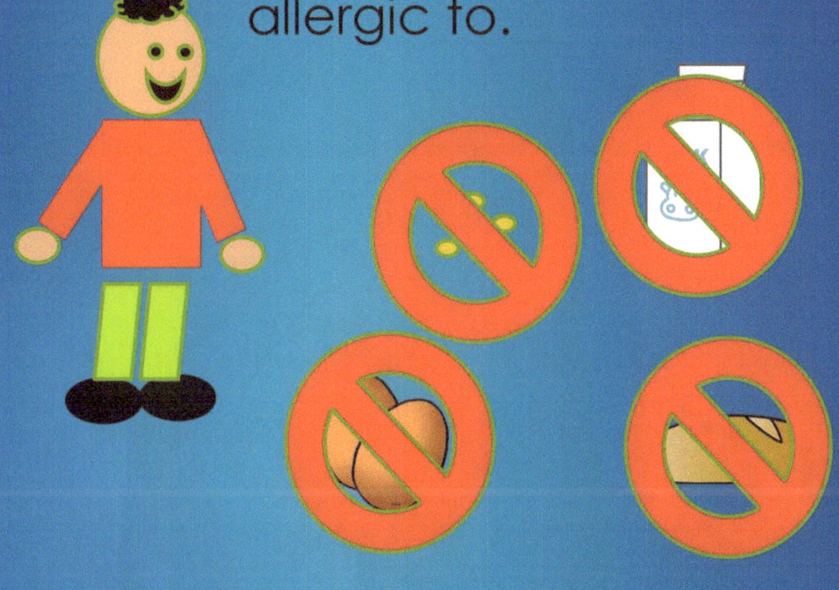

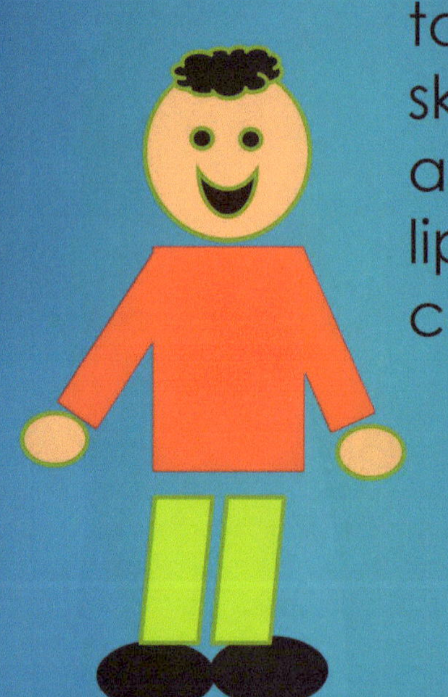

If Alex eats a food he is allergic to, he gets itchy skin, stomach aches, swollen lips, and a bad cough.

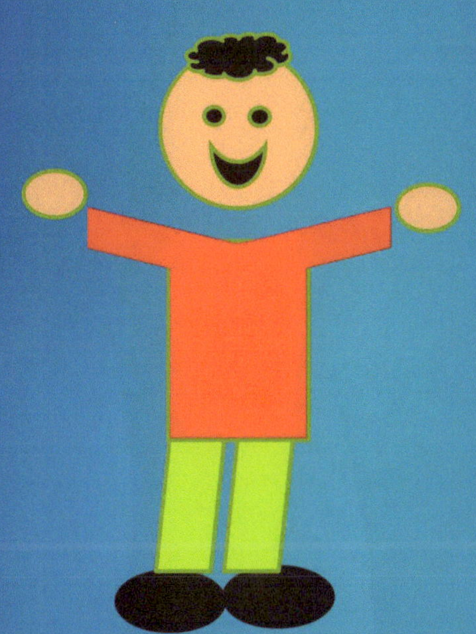

Alex likes to eat and wants to someday be able to eat all the foods...

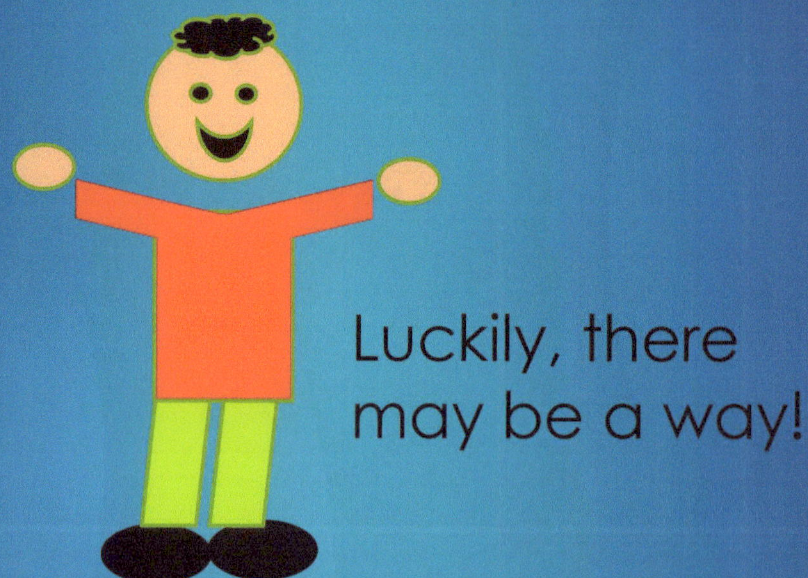

Luckily, there
may be a way!

He has to go to a special doctor, an allergist, who can teach his body how to NOT REACT when he eats something he is allergic to…

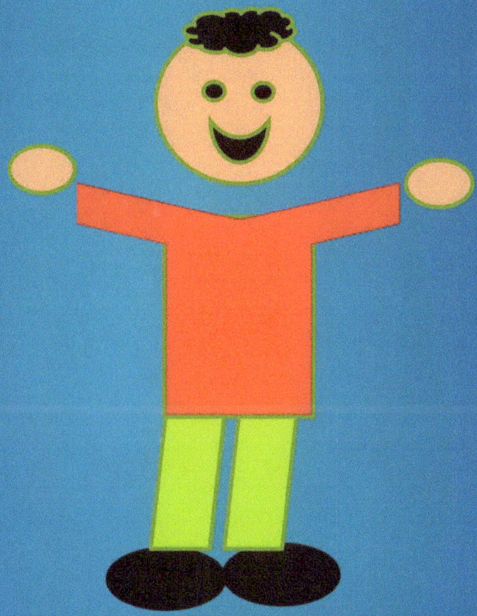

...AND DO SOMETHING CALLED ORAL IMMUNOTHERAPY, OR OIT FOR SHORT

During OIT, the doctor gives you a teeny, tiny amount of food that you are allergic to. So tiny, that your immune system doesn't see it and doesn't notice it.

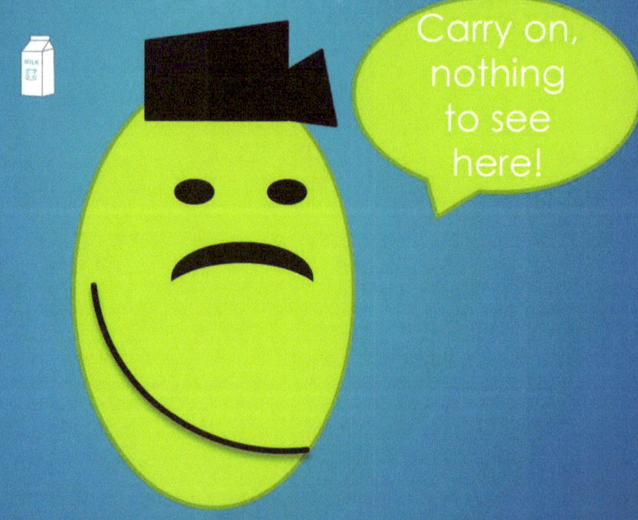

The doctor gives you a dose
to take every day
with special instructions you
have to follow.
Do you want to know what
they are?
Alex can show you his
instructions.

Alex's Doctor instructed:
First, you have to eat a little, then take your dose,
then relax and play <u>quietly</u> so that your heart does not speed up:
    you can't run around,
    you can't go swimming,
    you can't jump around.
You can only do things like read, watch TV, build with blocks…

Alex's doctor told him:
You MUST follow the rules.
If you don't follow the rules, you could get sick.
You have to take your dose every day or your immune system will not learn.
You can only do what your doctor tells you to do.

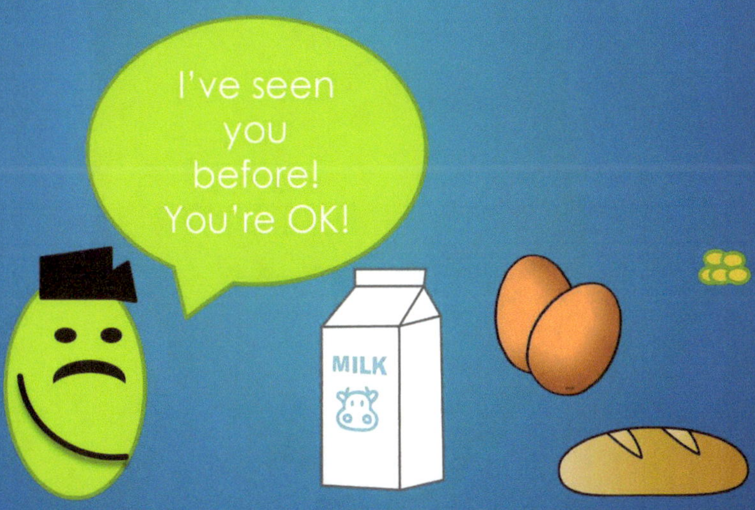

As time goes on, your dose will increase.
And if your dose is high enough, and your doctor says its ok, you may be able to eat your allergic food as much as you want!

Remember to always follow your doctor's instructions!

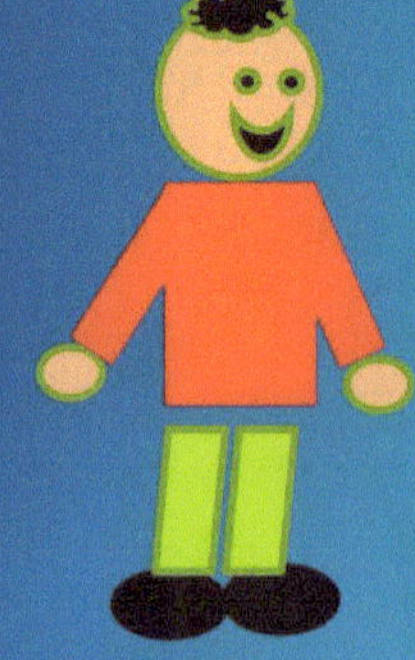

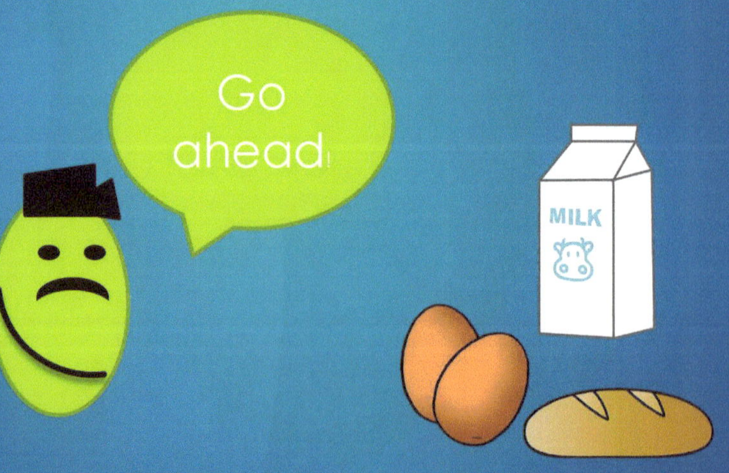

Alex shared his OIT rules
with you....

...... What are your OIT rules?

www.ingramcontent.com/pod-product-compliance
Lightning Source LLC
Chambersburg PA
CBHW040933110726

48006CB00001B/169